SLEEP WELL

Treatment to sleep and have a deep sleep, regulating your biorhythms, as well as a natural remedy to have a deep sleep. Overcome your sleep problems, renew your body and mind.

Ayuno Fitness

CREDITS

Copyright 2020 for **Ayuno Fitness**

Table of Contents

INTRODUCTION

The vast majority of people know about the enormous benefits that sleep gives us such as, more energy, more concentration capacity, better metabolism, less accumulation of fat in our body, etc., given many circumstances that usually happen in our daily life do not allow us to carry out a quality of sleep that we should have. There are more and more demands in your day-to-day life and it becomes more difficult to achieve those 8 hours of sleep you need. That's why we are going to recommend these strategies that will improve your quality of sleep and make those 6 hours or 5 hours that you normally sleep, worth as if they were 8 hours or more.

CHAPTER 1

Strategies for sleeping deeply in the rem phase

Your body is incredibly sensitive to the light that exists while you are sleeping, normally you were exposed more than 2000 years ago, to a situation where there was sun and that was the only time your brain received light, that happened from sunrise to sunset, and after that there was no other type of light. Since the appearance of electric light, man has slept an average of 2 to 3 hours less per day than before, and it is the great cause of a great many diseases that are beginning to appear in greater intensity, such as Alzheimer's and other similar types of dementia.

What impacts of light do we normally have on our daily lives?

The most common is blue light. Blue light is what you receive from your cell phone screen, computer, television, device, etc., and that in your brain causes more activity at the occipital lobe level that will take some time in your body to stop acting, this means that during 2 hours your brain at the occipital lobe level will be excited and active, this also means less quality of sleep when you are in your sleep hours.

So how do we go about changing this?

Here we share with you the following strategies to achieve a deep and beneficial sleep.

Sleeping in absolute darkness

Absolute means that no light enters the room you are sleeping and it is not as difficult as it seems, it is scientifically proven that if you point a laser (normal laser used to aim) at the skin of a person who is sleeping, their brain activity increases, that's how sensitive we are to light.

Devices off

The first and most advisable thing in this type of cases is not to use the cell phone, nor the computer 2 hours before you go to sleep, as this usually doesn't happen, put the filter night mode that is a blue light filter that what it does is decrease the amount of light with blue and violet spectrum that reaches your eyes, that is the one that more modifies what in your biological clock is called circadian cycle that generates that alteration modification that makes you feel awake. Nowadays, cell phones and computers have the night mode filter, except for some devices. When you make this function appear on your device you will notice that the screen turns a little sepia in color and that is perfect, since it will reduce the impact of light notably and obviously the final result will not be the same if you do not use the screen completely, but it is a good method that you can carry out, in addition it is something sustainable that will not take you much effort to carry out therefore applicable.

Temperature

The second thing has to do with the temperature you have in the room you are going to sleep, normally the temperature in which we usually sleep that has to do with our comfort is much higher than what our body really needs to fall asleep, today there are studies that show that people with insomnia refractory to bone treatment that even with medication were not able to fall asleep correctly, they achieve it through the use of helmets or devices that go in the head that cool the head because they lower the brain activity, the good news of all this is that you do not need to apply any of this, what you need to do is to put the temperature of the room you're sleeping at the ideal temperature to fall asleep which is much lower than people think, today it is estimated to be exactly about 18 degrees in general, the ideal and we recommend it is between 15 and 20 degrees and is as simple as putting the air conditioning at less than 20 degrees and if I have cold cover me with more sheets, because anyway the cold is going to get to the head and decrease the amount of brain activity that is, facilitating sleep and also this is very beneficial to people who often wake up during the night because the drop in brain activity forced by the temperature of the environment helps you have a deeper sleep and wake up less times during the night.

Meditation

This is a very common activity and that brings multiple benefits and that many people knowing about these, they do not perform, and is any type of meditation or strategies such as prayer or any practice of appreciation that you want to implement, to help you lower brain activity, calm down and this can be done in 20 or 10 minutes or as long as you want, keep this in mind always, no matter what strategies you use, if you do exercises of gratitude, transcendental meditation or whatever you want to do, the important thing is that you do it daily so you can develop the habit in your brain. Normally people say that they don't do it because they don't have time or because they are going to sleep only 6 hours, and 20 minutes less would imply a bad dream, the reality of this is not like that and today it is convenient for you 100 times to do the exercises or practices that you consider that serve you to sleep more deeply in spite of the fact that you sleep 20 minutes less, because the level of quality of sleep that you are going to have is going to be much greater and this is due to a decrease in the frequency of the cerebral activity that is measured in waves. Normally most human beings are functioning with beta waves that are between 15 to 30 Hertz and in reality, to fall asleep we should be lowering our brain activity each time and reducing the amount of speed at which those electromagnetic waves that activate our brain are given. Normally this happens from beta, first alpha, then to delta and deeper with theta waves which are the slowest in brain activity. Obviously, the more you practice meditation, the more results you will get, but it is always something that will give you quality sleep.

These following recommendations instead of sleep quality have more to do with the quality of waking up which will allow you during the day to feel fresh, awake, feel that you had a good quality of sleep thanks to training your circadian cycle, the latter meaning the day and night cycle for your brain.

Too many people have disturbed this cycle, that the difficulty of sleep passes specifically by this topic, by a bad circadian cycle, so much so that there are people who improve quickly with 2 or 3 recommendations that we will share with you below.

Drink half a liter of water

The first is that when you wake up there is a sensation that everyone usually experiences and that is "thirst". Thirst is the first sensation you experience since you wake up, this means that your body during the night of sleep is dehydrated and you need a great hydration at that moment, the first advice is to drink at least half a liter of water, if you have some kind of ritual such as drinking coffee or other drinks, the first thing you consume is water so that your body works properly, because if you drink coffee for example that is an adrenaline pump for your adrenal glands, which means a lot of stress for them, because with dehydration caffeine acts more proportionally, then this is not something positive for you, because you are living from reserves, you are using energy from reserves as if it was your normal day energy and this in the long run brings many conflicts not only with the circadian cycle but with the energy levels throughout the day. To recapitulate, you drink a half liter of water when you wake up and your body already recovers from this hydration factor incurred during the night.

Exposure to natural light

The second thing you should do to this is, if you were the night of sleep exposed to absolute darkness, what you should do is expose yourself to natural light during the day, this is recreated in the following way very easily for example, I get up, I drink my glass of water my half liter and you do it in front of the window, if it is summer you could go out to the balcony and in winter you could be glued to the window while you are drinking your water at the same time receiving the natural light that gives you in the face and body, this tells my brain "I am awake" and begins the circadian cycle working normally and through this process the cycle is retrained to be sleepy at night as it should be and to have a greater production of melatonin that will allow you to sleep more deeply.

Moderate physical activity

The third factor you have to take into account when you wake up is movement and exercise. Exercising does not mean that you have to start lifting weights as soon as you get up, although it would be extremely beneficial and it has been proven that it is one of the best times to exercise because it is the time when more neurotrophins are produced. The neurotrophins help to create new neurons, continuing with the exercise, it is necessary to understand the following thing, when it is recommended to make exercise when you get up and it is that while more movements you make as soon as you get up by more than a moderate movement, your body is going to understand that it is the moment to be awake and to modify all those physiological patterns that came supporting during the dream. Think about this, what you normally find is that you arrive at work and all the people are asleep, because they are asleep if they have been awake for 1 hour, because these physiological patterns that happen as soon as you wake up are not interrupted in any way, but are interrupted in a natural way your body continues to think physiologically that you are sleeping. So, with these simple tips you will be able to make your quality of sleep increase dramatically, you are not changing your life, they do not require a great amount of willpower, they are very simple to carry out and you can transform those 6 hours of sleep you have into about 8 hours in terms of quality of sleep.

CHAPTER 2

More strategies for better quality of sleep and better sleep

Avoid consumption of drinks with caffeine

Avoid doing this 6 hours before sleeping. Consume tea, guarana, coffee, pre-workouts and any kind of substance that increases adrenaline in your body. If your case is to train at night or if you work until late at night and want to be with energy to perform, you may feel like drinking high amounts of caffeine, the problem is this, that when you go to sleep your nervous system is activated mainly by the sympathetic route that is linked to adrenaline, noradrenaline, dopamine, that will prevent you from efficiently releasing melatonin and serotonin, which are the molecules that will allow you to achieve a long sleep of 7.8, 9 hours and above all to enter the rem sleep phase, which is the deep sleep phase where you release growth hormones. Then if you are of the people who sleep at 11 o'clock at night or more, try that at 5 o'clock in the afternoon you avoid the consumption of some food with high doses of caffeine that increases the adrenaline in the organism.

Regulating biorhythms

Biorhythms are the processes by which the body depending on the time of day activates certain hormonal metabolic processes and from there the body depending on whether it is day or night produces release of dopamine and adrenaline at times of day to be very active and goes on to release serotonin and melatonin at other times of day to be quiet, lower brain activity and especially allow a deeper sleep. If you want to improve the functionality of your biorhythms, we recommend that you do intermittent fasting depending on the degree of adherence you have with this practice, so you can activate the release of adrenaline, noradrenaline and dopamine because your body will feel the need to start, to activate, to go in search of the daily tasks you do and the sympathetic system will be activated. We also recommend if you are going to do sport that you do it in the morning hours, to regulate your biorhythms because at night your body mainly has to rest and will go to sleep activated, so try to make aerobic or anaerobic sport in the morning and that your first intake is ideally at 10 or 11 in the morning, should be high in protein and fat, because proteins promote the entry of tyrosine in your brain and thanks to tyrosine you increase the production of dopamine, so if you also want to improve the balance of your biorhythms you can incorporate 1000 to 1500 milligrams of L - tyrosine on an empty stomach to promote this release of dopamine. When you're getting to the last hours of the day you can use tools to let your body know that it's time to sleep and it's time for your serotonin is high and especially your melatonin, which is the hormone that is released by your pineal gland that will allow you to induce sleep. This is achieved by doing sport in the morning or by taking in carbohydrates some days at night, which will allow tryptophan to enter the brain and release serotonin. If you are a person who tries to sleep deeper, eating a legume, a sweet potato, a brown rice, will allow the tryptophan to enter better in the brain, have more serotonin and sleep deeper, in the end it is about balance.

No late-night dinners

We recommend that your dinner is not very abundant, many cardiovascular disorders, cerebrovascular, increased blood pressure, adrenaline, can occur throughout the night, often occur because late at night people are eating, is eating foods high in trans fats, especially when they are high in glycemic index and the person lies down with intestinal work, releasing hydrochloric acid, which generates gastritis and reflux all night generating discomfort, not being able to enter the rem sleep phase, also generating abdominal distention. This causes the organism to work at an intestinal level, at a hepatic level, at a lymphatic level all night long and in addition to that it cannot exercise the function of detoxifying because it is working to be able to absorb the nutrients, with which it lacks the capacity at night to detoxify, with which later you wake up tired, with a scratchy, white, swollen eye and this usually happens to many people who are eating late at night and after half an hour or even less are going to bed trying to sleep, and even if they manage to sleep it is most likely not a quality sleep.

The body is prepared for the 6 to 7 pm is our last intake and that is that in many countries like England, Holland, among others, apply this mentioned, in Latin countries we are used to eating late at night and try to sleep immediately, which generates problems when it comes to sleep. If you're one of those who are used to that, we recommend that you go down the hours that is your last intake so you can get a deep sleep and quality.

Sunbathing

It is very important that the levels of vitamin D are controlled in your organism, the hormonal levels, the activity of your nervous system, the liberation of serotonin etc., is very linked to the amounts of vitamin D, in addition when your organism is able to recognize in the early hours of the day like 9 or 10 in the morning only to a sun exhibition by about 15 minutes at least, the photons that are going to enter by our eye are going to generate a stimulus, at level of our pineal gland, hypothalamus, etc., to know that at 12 hours it is time to start producing serotonin and melatonin, this is a simpler tool for the body to start balancing the biorhythms again. Expose yourself in the morning only 15 minutes walking in short stretches exposed to the sun, do not do it with sunglasses so that the body recognizes that it is daytime and at approximately 12 hours is when the entry of the night should coincide with the descent of the photons from the sun with the rise of serotonin and melatonin. Now if you are one of those people who lives where the sun does not shine, or works from early in the morning in a closed place until the night, we recommend that in the months of winter or at the time that the sun does not shine then you ingest some supplement of vitamin D, so that you can control at least the impact that it can generate at level of hormonal system and to neuronal system and the low concentration of vitamin D in your organism.

Sleeping in absolute darkness

As we had mentioned before, sleeping in the dark makes our organism regulate its biorhythms since it lets itself be carried away by external conditioners to regulate the biorhythms, because when it is daytime the organism knows it is daytime and generates hormonal modulations, adrenaline releases to act on our day, and when our organism knows it is nighttime the release of serotonin, melatonin and all the molecules destined to have a deep sleep or rem phase takes place. If you are a person who has devices in the room where you sleep and the light of these is giving you to your body, this will cost you to enter into sleep and will cost your body to recognize that it is time to enter deep sleep, also if you are a person who has jobs as a police officer, nurse, watchman or night work in which you are required to be awake until late at night or even early morning and sleep in the morning either 2 or 3 in the morning, then try to cover any ray of light in your room, which is total darkness in your room, because if you leave open spaces where light enters either artificial or natural light, your body will think it's time to wake up and your sleep is half, making it impossible to have a dream in rem phase, which will generate the problems already mentioned, then the hours you go to sleep are 8 hours or more, which are in total darkness.

Zero electronic devices

Not to be exposed to mobile devices before sleeping or to electronic devices, since we are exposed to radiation that alters the functions of the brain and that has great scientific evidence. If you are one of the people who sleeps with the cell phone next to you, this will cause you to have a bad quality of sleep, that is why we recommend you to get rid of the mobile devices 1 or 2 hours before sleeping, these strategies will help you to have a good sleep.

Supplements

All the shared strategies, should serve you to improve your biorhythms, to improve the release of melatonin and serotonin, to improve the impact you can have with the devices making them much smaller, besides that with these tools you can have a better sleep, repair and balance. But if you are one of those people who is constantly struggling with sleep problems, if you are one of those people who after trying many natural tools in the end you do not get results, you still have insomnia, even taking pills you do not manage to sleep, then you can take supplements, and guided by a professional little by little you can go retiring the pills directed to the dream in case these taking pills for the dream at the moment, because the pills allow you to sleep but not of physiological form for that reason in many occasions you wake up with the hurt body, tired, annoyed, with legañas, with the cloudy mind, etc. , what we are interested in is that you have a balanced sleep, endogenous by its own mechanisms, here we share with you the supplements we recommend.

Melatonin along with Gaba, melatonin should ideally be sublingual or in the form of transdermal cream, any doctor can do it in a masterful formula 5 milligrams per night between 3 and 5 milligrams, or even orally, but in many occasions the bioavailability is not the same, and if it can be combined with about 500 milligrams of Gaba.

The Gaba will allow you to lower your alert state, it will allow your nervous system to turn off the alarm signal. These two supplements together will make you sleep and also have a rem sleep, if you are a person who performs sports, you have a day full of activities that you have to be constantly on the move, and if you do not eat properly, you may lack minerals such as calcium and magnesium which are minerals that allow us to relax muscles, And you are one of those people who neglect too much their diet, so before sleeping try to consume 800 to 1200 milligrams of calcium along with 400 milligrams of magnesium and also use calcium, and throughout the week from 7 000 units to 10 000 units of vitamin D to promote the bioavailability of calcium. These minerals taken before sleeping, will make your nervous system more relaxed and your muscles to relax. Since your nervous system is activated at night and from there appear shocks, pain in the body, cervical etc., you can also take some B complex, vitamin B6 that promotes the activity of tryptophan, to release serotonin and melatonin. Here we will make an aside, if you are a person who has malnutrition, you will have the nervous system activated, you will have the sympathetic nervous system which is the one that releases, adrenaline noradrenaline, dopamine very activated throughout the day because the body continues to seek nutrients, then it is ideal to balance your nutrition and if you are a sportsman with much more reason, with amino acids and essential oils, since there have been many cases of people who did not sleep at night and by a simple inclusion of 20 grams of essential amino acids throughout the day to cover the essential needs of the muscles has allowed the body to feel that it is not time 24 hours a day to look for food and has allowed itself to relax and at night the body has lowered the alarm signal, so to what is recommended with the sleep supplements also add the recommended amino acids so you can better optimize your body.

Adaptogens

If you are one of those people with a lot of stress, who stop working and also have a lot of physical as well as mental wear and tear, the ideal that we recommend here is that you consume adaptations such as ashwaganndha. If you have hormonal defects, if you are a man over 50 or a woman who has already gone through menopause, talk to your doctor, urologist in the case of men and gynecologist in the case of women to see the levels of testosterone in the case of men and estradiol and progesterone in the case of women, because these processes of hormonal descent usually imply a lot of imbalance in the dreams, especially if you are a woman with menopause where that impact of 6 to 12 months where your organism has stopped releasing estrogen can alter your dream too much, for that reason it speaks with your doctor and it values a hormonal replacement.

No pressure to fall asleep

When you pressure yourself to sleep you generate anxiety and impetus to force yourself to sleep, you also generate a state of mental alertness, for example if after your normal day you watch a movie late at night to disconnect and without realizing it you fall asleep because you are without that pressure to want to sleep immediately, But the moment you try to sleep again you generate that state of mental alertness and it will be even more difficult to sleep, so we recommend that you do not try to fight to fall asleep, it is best to accept that the time will come when you fall asleep that will allow your mental alert, your adrenaline in your body to drop and without realizing it you will go into a deep sleep.

Let's remember that sleep is very important for the functioning of your hormones, for your immune system, for the functioning of your brain, for your emotional state, for living in society in a happy way and without quality of sleep all these areas mentioned are going to decline considerably.

CHAPTER 3

MELATONIN THE SLEEP HORMONE

The big problems in our advanced society are sleep problems, so in this chapter we will share with you the knowledge about what melatonin is and how you can use it to get a deep sleep-in rem phase that is very beneficial to you.

Melatonin and biorhythms

When we talk about the tools to improve your health, we especially talk about tools that are going to improve your biorhythms, and whenever we talk about biorhythms we have to talk about getting the right amount of sleep, normally sleep should be before 12 noon, which ideally should be between 7 and 9 hours and should be deep enough to reach the rem phase, which gives you the following benefits like regenerate the body, hormones such as growth hormone are released, substances, molecules and molecular pathways are released that allow you to wake up in a good mood, with high energy levels, to be able to perform better in your day to day and overcome the difficulties that are presented, and while using the natural tools to sleep properly will be ideal to restore your health in a comprehensive manner. This is where melatonin comes into play, this great hormone that is now much more easily found in herbalists, in supplement stores, in pharmacies and here we will solve the most common questions about this hormone.

The first thing we have to understand is that the hormone melatonin is released in the pineal gland and is released as a consequence of having a good functioning of your biorhythms. We have talked about that around 10 to 11 in the morning you should expose yourself to the photons of the solar light, activate yourself in the morning, so that the organism feels the sufficient activity of the sympathetic nervous system, the liberation of catecholamines, of dopamine, of adrenaline, the exposure of those photons to the sun, so that the retina captures those photons and that information reaches the supraquiasmatic nucleus which is a small area of 10 000 neurons of the hypothalamus and that area informs your pineal gland, that approximately 10 to 12 hours after the exposure to the photons of the sun you can begin to release melatonin, that will allow you to fall into a deep sleep at 10 to 11 o'clock at night.

Any situation that affects the correct functioning of your biorhythms will also diminish your quality of sleep, for example, because you get up late, because you have a bad diet, because you work in the dark early in the morning, because you drink a lot of coffee at night, because you arrive with a lot of stress from work, because you train late at night and this generates hyperactivity in your nervous system, maybe you are on an extreme ketogenic diet or you have an extreme caloric deficit, all these variants affect our biorhythms and when it comes to synthesizing in a coherent way the concentrations you need in your nervous system of melatonin, it does not reach the necessary level for you to sleep correctly and develop all the immunological, nervous, intestinal routes etc. , that at night has to develop in the right way. It is important to know that melatonin is manufactured from tryptophan which has to be transformed into serotonin which is the neurotransmitter that we know is important for mental peace, to better face stress, that's why we have to take into account that in a diet where there is a lack of carbohydrates there will be a deficit in terms of the entry of tryptophan through the blood-brain barrier to the interior of the nervous system and there can be a deficiency of serotonin and a deficit in terms of the production of melatonin at night. That is why if you are one of those people who fast intermittently from one day to the next, do a lot of sport, eat an extreme ketogenic diet and are not adapted to these new strategies, to fats as a main source of energy, it could be that, weeks after starting all these tools, you will be having sleep problems. If you want to have a good synthesis of melatonin in the concentrations that are necessary for you, it is important and necessary that all the tools mentioned above are carried out in an integral way, consistently according to the context and remember to include in your healthy diet carbohydrates 2 to 3 nights in the week and if you train you can include after your workout at 6 to 7 pm an inclusion of carbohydrates such as sweet potato, tuber, brown or white rice, always remember that not killing the carbohydrate kills the amounts you eat that make them accumulate as glycogen reserves. These hydrates will help us to facilitate the entry of tryptophan, the synthesis of serotonin and finally of nocturnal melatonin, which will have many positive consequences on your performance, on your neuronal system, on your emotional system, on your immune system, etc.

Functions of Melatonin

Melatonin allows us to relax enough to fall into deep sleep, thanks to melatonin allows the muscles of your body to relax and this is essential because it does not serve you to train 3 hours throughout the day if at night you are not able to relax your muscles (this is an example, we do not recommend training for more than 1 hour unless you are a high performance sportsman) since by not relaxing, you are not exposing yourself to the necessary oxygenation, to the hormones that have to be released to facilitate hypertrophy, etc.

Melatonin has hormonal functions, it has immunomodulatory functions, melatonin has a great influence on the immunological functions, on the correct release of lymphocytes, macrophages, on the immune adaptation that the body must have to autoimmune processes, to exposure to parasites, etc., melatonin has been shown to generate an immune modulation at the intestinal level, that is why it has been observed that the intestine is capable of releasing small fractions of melatonin and people who include melatonin in their intake of supplements and have gastrointestinal problems, chronic diseases, ulcerative colitis, have been able to observe some favorable evolution after this incorporation of melatonin externally.

Melatonin has antioxidant functions; melatonin can have up to 200/300 times more antioxidant power than resveratrol. It has also been observed that there are small amounts of melatonin in the mitochondria, within the mitochondria is known that there are many substances derived from oxygen, many free radicals which generates long-term mitochondrial problems, mitochondrial diseases, myopia, certain tumors that have problems in the functioning of mitochondria and hence it is speculated that this small amount of melatonin that is within the mitochondria acts as an antioxidant.

One very important function that you should keep in mind is the best insulin sensitivity and to avoid hepatic neoglucogenesis, this means that throughout our lives and from the age of 35 to 40 especially in Western society with so many bad habits, with so much consumption of processed foods, high consumption of refined sugars, lack of physical activity, sedentary life, emotional conflicts and biorhythm alterations, a person from 35 to 40 years old with some of the above mentioned cases is more susceptible and more predisposed to all the metabolic problems that revolve around the metabolic syndrome and type 2 diabetes, the alterations of the lipid profile, elevated triglycerides, alterations of the cholesterol levels, greater blood coagulation, cardiovascular accidents, immunological alterations, alteration of the body composition, greater increase of the abdominal fat, greater increase of the chronic inflammation of low degrees, all these problems are problems derived from the metabolic syndrome, that has like base that peripheral resistance to the insulin and a hepatic neoglucogenesis, that means that it produces and it releases to the blood glucose plasma, which generates hyperglycemias to us.

Melatonin improves the sensitivity and flexibility of the peripheral receptors to insulin, which allows our pancreas not to have to release so much insulin when faced with carbohydrate loads on a daily basis, because this insulin will link the peripheral receptors to insulin much better, and thanks to melatonin, hepatic neoglycogenesis, which can generate nocturnal hyperglycemia, is avoided. A small amount of melatonin has been shown to improve sensitivity to insulin, hepatic neoglucogenesis, predisposition to type 2 diabetes and all these pathologies of the metabolic syndrome.

If you travel outside of your country where the time difference is 7 hours or more and that prevents you from sleeping the first days or even weeks, melatonin comes into action as the fundamental supplement to be able to expose yourself and quickly adapt to that jetlag, that time difference that makes the first days unable to adapt to the biorhythms of the new country where you are a small amount of 1 and 2 milligrams can serve you so that from day one you can adapt to the new schedules that apply.

Safe dosage of how melatonin should be ingested

Melatonin is mainly found in tablets of 1.8 / 1.9 mg in the supplement market, but you can take it safely between 0.5 / 5 mg per day, that is the dose we recommend at the end depends on the tolerance of each person, the bioavailability of melatonin that is generated within your body, the detoxification you generate from the residue etc., each person has different types of sensitivity to this hormone, we recommend that you should try it initially between 0.5mg to 5mg.

Melatonin has synergies with magnesium and Gaba, we recommend that you consume between 200 to 400 mg of magnesium and about 500 to 600mg of Gaba can be an ideal combination to go to sleep combined with melatonin.

Melatonin Side Effects

The tolerance of melatonin is very high, studies have been done with up to 3000 mg, the usual dose we recommend between 0.5 mg to 5 mg, but there have been studies where people have come to consume between 3000 mg to 4000mg and no significant side effects have been observed. There are endocrinologists, geriatricians, oncologists who give their patients in special cases between 200 mg a day, and there have also been other professionals who recommend patients with certain pathologies where they are given between 50 and 100mg of melatonin daily due to its high antioxidant content, so don't worry about this hormone intoxication, but in certain cases if, for example, young children between 6 and 8 months we don't recommend any type of melatonin dose, there is no study in babies, biorhythms at that age are not consolidated, but anyway we recommend you to talk to your pediatrician, because there have been studies that determine that in cases of children with neurological problems, with autism, with attention deficit, with hyperactivity it was observed that there is certain improvement in their behavior due to the antioxidant capacity of melatonin to neuronal effects, in this type of cases cerebral melatonin is used, this is vehiculated with liposomes that have greater adherence by certain brain areas and it has been observed in cases of children with autism that when exposed to melatonin at certain doses it does not give them side effects and above all the most remarkable thing is that their behavior improves. If you have a child who is not in these cases mentioned, we do not recommend using melatonin until the person is 23 to 25 years old onwards, because at 25 years old people have a considerable decline of melatonin by the pineal gland, in addition at 25 years old there is not much risk in terms of negative feedback, this means that by ingesting external melatonin you stop producing melatonin naturally, since at 25 years old we do not release much of this hormone.

If you don't sleep well between the ages of 18 and 22, you should check your stress or anxiety levels, the nervousness that is generated every day, if you lead a very sedentary life, the activities that you do every day, you stop in front of the computer or mobile devices for a long time and your biorhythms are diminished, for that reason use the shared tools so that as soon as possible you correct those errors that lead you to a bad quality of sleep.

Another side effect is that you overdose or take it too late, around 2 or 3 in the morning. This will make you wake up the next day tired, irritated, and with reduced concentration.

Alteration in the levels of sexual hormones, these cases usually occur in athletes or people who consume more than 10 mg per day. From 10mg onwards, melatonin generates a decrease in GNRH, which is the hypothalamic gonadotropin-releasing hormone that tells the pituitary gland to release LH and FCH, which are the pituitary hormones that will tell your gonads, ovaries if you are a woman, and testicles if you are a man, to release the sexual Mormons that will enable our sexual functions.

We have melatonin in very high concentrations in our pineal gland until approximately 9 or 10 years of age, from that age a decline of this hormone is generated since it generates the birth of the sexual hormones in the boys and in the girls, by the so abrupt fall of these concentrations of melatonin, the pineal gland stops releasing that melatonin and there is an activation at the level of the hypothalamus and pituitary gland in terms of the release of hormones that are going to favor the birth of the hormonal explosion whether you are a man or a woman, for example the periods of menstruation in women, The release of testosterone in men and everything happens by a decline and fall to very low levels of melatonin, so if you ingest high levels of melatonin between 10, 15 ,20 mg to more a day is very possible that your levels of GNRH decrease, if you are man that your levels of testosterone decrease and if you are woman that your levels of estrogen and progesterone may fall and you lose your period, This has been observed in athletes, also in women with very low percentage of body fat and therefore do not sleep are very hyperactive and therefore take much of melatonin to sleep, melatonin in the doses we recommend between 0. 5 to 5 mg will not give you problems with your sex hormones.

Melatonin has anticoagulant effects in your blood, if you are a person who is on medication and take medications such as heparin, with any type of anticoagulant, talk to your doctor who will review the dosage of melatonin and recommend that you take it or if in your case it is not necessary to take it because it would generate adverse effects, in this case you could take other supplements such as magnesium, Gaba, and passion flower, but we recommend that you talk to your doctor or cardiologist if you take this type of medication.

CHAPTER 4

Ritual to help you sleep soundly

As a last strategy we will share with you our ritual so you can sleep like a baby.

1. It consists of going to bed at 11 o'clock at night to enter the rem phase of deep sleep from 12 o'clock onwards. It has been proven that 12 to 3 o'clock gives a very deep regeneration and produces greater amounts of growth hormones and testosterone.

2. At 7 o'clock we finish working, we turn off the mobile devices and go for a walk, if you live near the sea much better, but you can also do it to the square or place with nature that is with a measured silence, also have the precautions of the case in case your city is something dangerous, always safeguard our integrity, let's continue with this walk keep in mind not to carry mobile devices and disconnect from work, you enjoy that walk, relax, do not think about business, do not think about relationships, unless you do it as a couple try that each one remains silent while walking.

3. When you get home take a hot bath and apply epsom salt to your tub. Epsom salts contain magnesium and magnesium is a very important mineral that promotes muscle relaxation and also the relaxation of the nervous system among its many benefits and discoveries about this great mineral. In fact, several studies show that the correct way to

obtain maximum benefits from this mineral is not through diet or supplementation, but through the skin.

4. Read a book of fiction so that your mind continues with that active disconnection that you had from work, study, etc., that activity that makes your mind alert, that is why this book that we also recommend will help you relax. If you don't feel like reading, you can watch comedy videos, but do it on devices that eliminate white light, white light affects the production of melatonin and makes it difficult for us to fall asleep as we mentioned before. That's if you take into account that the other devices are off, such as cell phones, televisions, etc.

5. If you cannot take a bath in hot water and epsom salt, you can apply magnesium oil.

6. Before you go to bed, take this magic infusion that will help you sleep properly and have a deep sleep-in rem phase, is to mix 2 tablespoons of organic honey plus 2 tablespoons of apple cider, if you like you can also mix it with a little hot water and an infusion of lime blossom, lemon verbena, chamomile, but remember that the most important ingredients are quality honey and apple cider vinegar.

Many people with insomnia who have tried our ritual have benefited from it because they have been able to enter their deep sleep-in rem phase and be able to access the benefits that sleep brings.

Keep in mind to apply each strategy shared in this book, no doubt apart from our magic ritual, each strategy is designed to achieve deep sleep access to the benefits of this and regulate your biorhythms, if even so the improvements have been remarkable, but you want the effect is faster, then apply our magic sleep ritual, we assure you that you will sleep deeply.

CHAPTER 5

The power of meditation

We live in a world where it is more and more complex and where there are also more people with bad moods, which makes everything make our mind feel anxious or depressed when that is not the natural state of any animal including human beings, all our sensory perceptions what we hear, what we see, What we smell are interpreted by our brain and we have specialized cells that transform these stimuli like sunlight, like someone's kiss into an electrical impulse that your brain will interpret and depending on areas of the brain you use more often and have more developed and trained in what interpretation and response you are going to give to all that. Basically, your brain builds the reality in which you live, so if you change the neural networks and this interpretation changes, would it change how I feel? And the answer is "yes" and that's basically what you have to do.

How do I change these areas that my brain uses? Y

How do I change this interpretation?

Here meditation plays a fundamental role since this great tool we can use to change all this.

Your brain trains as much as Cristiano Ronaldo for example who has a better shot than me because he trains for years, there are brain areas that besides defining how you are going to play soccer, define what interpretation you are going to give to what you are seeing or hearing, in the example of this sportsman they are better because his brain areas of motor coordination were trained to give better coordination, more strength, more skill etc., but the moral of all this is that they are trainable areas and what about the mood? are they also trainable? And the answer is "yes", imagine this situation for example, an ancestor of yours from more than 15 000 years ago is walking through the forest, he is gathering fences from a plant he found and he hears that suddenly a sound in the bushes, his brain at that moment can 2 options, you may decide that this stimulus is simply wind in the bushes or some small animal that poses no threat in the bushes where it could quietly gather more food and continue to gather that food to have more food later, and the other option where that sound represents a predator that may come to kill you for food, the predator's option is less likely, your ancestor's brain can generalize and assume that it is always wind and the sound it hears in the bushes but in the action in which it is indeed a predator your ancestor would be eaten by a predator, so your ancestor's brain chooses to assume that whenever it hears the sound in the bushes it has to assume that it is a predator, this kind of situations are called "false positives" where I always assume something is a threat when it is not necessarily, the problem is that for survival it makes much more sense to assume the false positive and think that there is always a real threat and run away because at most I will lose my berries but I will stay alive, this is the reason why when you have a problem your mind generates. Imagine the worst possible solution to the problem and exaggerate the potential risks of it to theoretically protect you, the problem is that we continue to be wired this way at the neural level to protect ourselves and survive even though those threats are no longer real, so if we come with a brain that comes factory wired that way how do we modify it?

And the answer is "training him to think differently" if I know that by nature, I come like this, it means that my happiness and tranquility depend effectively on training this kind of process, there will be people who are naturally more skilled than others in this kind of training, but we can all benefit from training our perception through meditation.

There are thousands and thousands of different types of meditations, all with the same objective which is to lower the excess of mental activity, to bring our brain a slower functioning more coordinated and less chaotic that does not generate less level of stress and less level of sensation of danger, this is not New Age theory, this we can measure in our brain, and we can measure the patterns of functioning of brain waves where people do more meditations, works longer because of a type of waves that are called alpha waves that make us more efficient, make us make fewer mistakes, make us have less sympathetic bone activity, less stress, less anxiety and give us a lot of health benefits, and comparing to those who do not meditate has more level of sympathetic activity and works more in beta waves that what they do is stress you more, make you more anxious or have less deep sleep and a lot of other consequences that tell you basically meditate.

The enormous majority of meditations propose something similar which is to concentrate on something external to lower the level of the internal dialogue of your mind, it can be a mantra, it can be to be attentive to your breathing or any other method that helps you to decrease the internal brain activity and our constant internal dialogue, you can use a mantra as they use in transcendental meditation, you can use techniques in which you are attentive to your breathing, the one you want, we will share with you a method that has worked for many people, it is used by Matthieu Ricard who is known as the happiest man in the world.

How do we meditate?

Sit in any position that is comfortable for you where your head is not resting on a surface, either on the wall or on the bed, or anywhere else, and if possible keep your spine straight without forcing it, this is simply so that you can improve your breathing technique when you are meditating and so that you do not fall asleep, There is no proven extra benefit to meditating in strange positions like the lotus, unless you have the flexibility to do so and enjoy assuming that posture, but choose the position in which you feel relaxed and where you feel you will not fall asleep.

What do I have to do during meditation?

Our brain is made to respond to these stimuli this means that the more external stimuli we have, the more brain activity we are going to have, that's why many types of meditation try to eliminate the external stimuli to less stimulus less response of my brain and that's why the enormous majority of the meditations usually close the eyes, usually they are in calm places where the sound is not going to interrupt my meditation, You can even listen to quiet music if you want to but you don't have to have any stimulus that is going to prevent the relaxation of the brain activity like a loud sound or like particularly marked lights, or people passing by you, none of these things are mandatory or mandatory just closing your eyes for example helps us to distract less from this process, What you are going to do in a normal meditation is to concentrate on your breathing, you are going to try to listen to your breath to be aware of the outside and have your senses try to pick up some information from the outside but at the same time you are going to breathe with an intensity in which you do not hear your breath, This is really paradoxical and it is trying to force your brain to listen to something from the outside to decrease the internal dialogue and at the same time have a calm enough breath to help you lower the brain activity, this basically puts your attention outside your brain, if I am breathing slowly and I don't get to listen to my breath but at the same time I am attentive to my breath.

How do I know if this process we call meditation is working?

Basically there are a lot of ways that the body communicates this lowering of the sympathetic activity, this lowering of the brain activity through relaxing the muscle tone, through lowering the breathing rate, through lowering the heart rate and if you are someone who enjoys doing experiments on his or her own and wants to see if indeed this meditation is having a result, you can meditate with a saturation meter and evaluate if your heart rate, if your breathing rate while you are meditating is going down, but it is really very easy to perceive in a meditation once I have been doing this for a while mentioned above, the physiological changes that are going to take place in your body when your body lowers the excessive brain activity and lowers the sympathetic activity of your autonomic nervous system.

How long do I have to meditate?

The average time of the different meditations should be 20 minutes, but if this is the first time you are going to meditate or the first time you are going to take meditation more seriously, start with 5 minutes that are easy for you to carry out, so that you start to generate the habit without it representing a burden or an effort that you have to make and that simply because it generates pleasure to you to do it.

How does a better emotional state feel?

Feeling it, in the same way that you train a motor skill by practicing it, you train an emotional skill by practicing it, you see many recommendations about gratefulness that are very wrong because they propose you to write a list of things that you are grateful for that for your brain do not mean anything because they have little intensity, then the proposal that we recommend is extremely simple, then take those 5 minutes that we recommended at the beginning about meditating when you are an initiate, take it to revive a circumstance of your life where it has given you enormous levels of gratitude, for example it can be the birth of a child, or the encounter with a loved one or the one you want but be clear about the following, revive it does not mean to see it in your mind, it means to feel again what you felt in that moment, then take your time to immerse yourself in that situation you are going to start seeing physical changes, changes in heart rate, changes in breathing rate, changes in muscle tone just like before but you are also going to notice a change in mood as you relive these positive situations of appreciation in your life, because your brain is not distinguishing whether it is happening here now or whether it is a memory that happened 10 years ago, What matters only are the sensations that you are feeling, basically your brain does not know that this is a memory and interprets it as if it were happening now, so as I do more and repeat it daily I will be developing these areas of the perception of gratitude that are transposed to your whole life, not to the five minutes that you do this practice. Here I recommend meditation programs so that you can realize that today what changes you can generate in your body and your state of mind with a meditation.

CONCLUSION

Apply every strategy we have shared with you, do not underestimate any of them because if you doubt, they will help you to have a deep sleep in the rem phase and regulate your biorhythms and as a consequence your health will improve a lot.

If you liked our book please leave a positive review, as it will help us continue working with greater quality.

If you want to sleep from now on, apply our ritual, if you have more serious problems, we will share our guide where you can solve that deep doubt.

Recommended programs:

_ EMPOWER YOUR BRAIN AND YOUR HEARING

https://e1756fy9mkpwhme7pf0z8u9wdr.hop.clickbank.net/

_ IMPROVE YOUR MEMORY

https://35f49k3eimwwjr19sireo6rv8n.hop.clickbank.net/

 SLEEP TO REVERSE DIABETES

https://3076aew7mmrs9wf85yxwbyas9d.hop.clickbank.net/

www.ingramcontent.com/pod-product-compliance
Lightning Source LLC
Chambersburg PA
CBHW071312130726
47997CB00007B/2527